I0829484

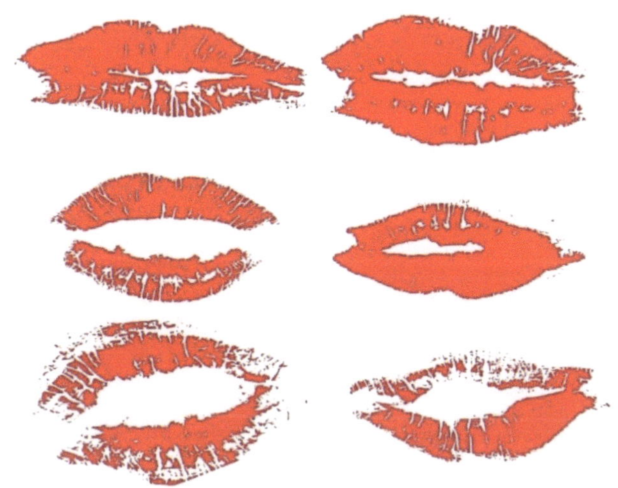

Love,

Love,

& More

Love!

A fresh perspective.

New thoughts

New Insight

Building Up Publishing ©2015

TOPICS

The next chapter is better!

Heart Breaker!

Decisions, Decisions, Decisions!

Lesson II

You are the Star

Wrong thinking about Love!

Changing Perceptions

Love!

Taking Inventory

I love engaging in discussions about love. Love is defined as tender affection for another person, sexual desire for another, or an affectionate concern for others. I wrote this book for people who have made mistakes in love and those who hate being in love. This book is about the journey of love. Love had taught me many lessons. As you read through this book think about experiences cause us to love more or love less. It doesn't matter if you are young, middle aged, or elder. Your ethnic background and gender does not matter because we are all born with a natural desire for love and relationships. Some people may not use the term love they may use the term happiness. This book does not focus on love as we see it in the movies or as we think about love as it relates to falling in love with a person but it is about a pure love and an learned ability to show it. I am talking about love on a deeper level. It is the love that exists among individuals who have lived long enough to experience heart break, betrayal, and heart ache. If you are a young person who is dating and learning please keep reading because you have picked up the right source because learning how to love is just like our natural development it takes time, experience, and knowledge.

In high school we are so positive about love and then we begin to experience hurt or the downside of dating and this begins to damper our views about love in our middle stages of life. But today we can learn that experience is a teacher and love is a friend. We can make love with others or make hate but love is my favorite subject because I have learned how to make it. It may seem strange but I enjoy love because love deals with the issues of the heart, and the heart is a special part of a person. The heart and mind functions together. Both need to be healthy and working properly. It is the will, emotions, and feelings of a person.

The heart has the ability to feel a wide range of emotions and we learn so much about ourselves as we deal with different situations in life. Dealing with the heart and emotions can also be chaotic and this is why I am so excited to talk about love and the different complex issues of the heart! I am opening up my heart to you with the hopes that this book opens up your heart to a love experience. Good or bad our love experience begin as a child.

Children's Ability to Love

According to scientific research parents play a significant role in the process and development of a child. Children do not know anything about love and they do not know anything about hate. If you see racism apparent in a child, he or she has learned it from their parents. Maybe some ideas come from television but when a child learns to mistreat others it is because he or she is raised in an environment that has either told him or showed him what to do. Children will learn how to love and hate based on what they learn from their environment. Learning involves speaking, interaction, and instilling ideas in children.

Children are like little people they will mimic the actions they see. A child can only give what he or she has been taught to give. The bible discloses that we must train up a child in the way he should go and when he is older he or she will not depart from it. This reveals unto me that children are in the process of being trained. It is up to parents to show their children love through tender kindness, nice words, and loving touches. Some people may think touch is silly. But some people spank their kids but never take the time to loving touch their face or hold them close. In a romantic relationship men and women bond through touch and children need loving touches just as much as adults. When I think about children who have been abandoned by a parent or both parents I foresee an adult(s) who will have problems in relationships. A parent who never learns how to love cannot teach their child how to love. If you are a parent like me then you realized the mistakes your parents made and most of us desire to do better than them. One must always watch the way we speak to others; how they treat others. Children watch behavior more than they listen words. It is odd that speaking is important and as an adult I understand and remember the things my mother said. As a child it went in one ear and out the other and most of the time I did what she said because I did not want a punishment. As adults we will live out the things we learned from our home environments. It is okay to admit to ourselves if we have been successful in love or not. Moving from a child to an adult we soon discover that our love experiences begin to change as we begin to date, mature, and experience life at different levels. Having an understanding about love can help people separate the good things learned as a child from the bad things that we learned in order to make our individual love experiences great. Some people learn from their mistakes. Some people are blind to their mistakes. Happiness is knowing how to forgive yourself. You were never perfect and if you had lots of failure like me learn to forgive yourself and anyone who

hurt you during a love experience. Admit the mistake and move on quickly.

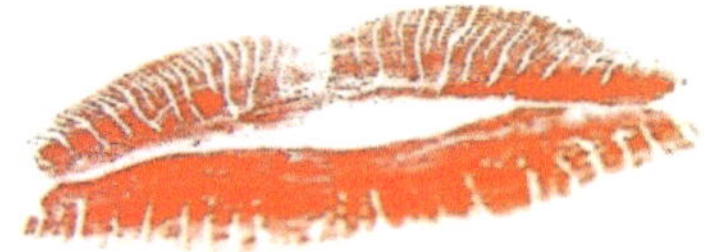

Natural Insight About love

New research has reveal what happens to the brain during a love experience. It may be surprising but research attacks the myth we all believed. What is the myth? It has been said that most people believe that when it comes to love they are dealing with the heart. But science tells us that we are not dealing with the heart but we are dealing with the brain. Customarily when we fall in love we feel knots in the stomach, anxiety, and an increase in heart rate, and a roller coaster ride of emotions when we are in the presence of the person we love. Even though these things are happening in the body we tend to believe that it is happening in our hearts but it is actually happening in the brain. When we think about love we must think rationally. We should not follow our feelings when in love. Think about it which makes more sense following feelings or logical smart choices. If you are in a relationship think about the silly things you did or said because you felt anger towards your mate, spouse, or friend. Following your feelings will destroy your relationship. A deeper love relationship means treating the person good and this takes using the brain. It means acting and enjoying the feelings but realizing that a good love experience is all about how you think, act, and respond to the other person as well as how they think, act, and respond to you. Love needs to be 20% feelings and 80% logic. I love Steve Harvey's book, *"Act like a Lady Think like a Man."* The book made me a little touchy but as I read through each chapter I realized that he was simply asking woman to stop throwing our brain away when we meet a man. He also revealed to men through his examples that it is immature to treat a woman like a rag you use one day and throw away the next. Men and women love differently and he encourages women to think like a man when dating. Experience has taught me to stop following my fleeting emotions and start implementing good judgement. If we are very honest we understand emotions leave and the reality is love for another person does not happen in two weeks despite feelings of love.

If your love is based upon the heart it will be an unstable questionable love; but when it is based upon the brain, we are empowered to make intelligent decisions about how we treat others. Enjoy the emotions and feelings but keep your brain turned on. Let the brain lead until the relationship is grounded then relax and enjoy the roller coaster of love.

The article also looked at brain chemistry. According to the article doctors looked at the brain chemistry of young people in love and researchers discovered that young people who confessed to have butterflies in their stomach when they were in contact with the person they love showed brain changes. The young people agreed to complete a brain scan; and the brain scan revealed that the individual's brain responded when they focused their thoughts on the object of their affection, and during this time a whole host of brain parts begin to light up.

The areas associated with dopamine and production parts of the brain lit up and this supported the hypothesis that just like chocolate love is addictive and it affects the brain. When it comes to marriage researchers have discovered that couples who idealized each other have the potential to remain happy for a long time. Oxytocin is called a love hormone and it is released in humans and animals during bonding. Maintaining the bond and protecting can make a married couple happy.

Now that we know that love operates in the brain and the importance of thinking on good things when it comes to those we love. We must remember that a host of different chemicals are released in the brain and that is why we feel like we are in love. Research has discovered some distinctions between men and women when it comes to sex, love, and the brain. Doctors have discovered that men have a sexual pursuit area that is 2.5 times larger than the one in the female brain; and surprisingly the male brain has stronger emotional reactions than the female brain, but research reveals that within seconds of the male having the emotion they are able to

change it within two to five seconds.

Agape Love

The supreme love of God reveals itself to man through his actions. His love is a wonderful thing and his love touches the very soul of man. It has nothing to do with romantic feelings. When I think about Agape love I think about actions. God has showed us his great love through Jesus Christ. "For God so loved the world he gave his only begotten son."

His love grips me deeply within and it causes me to ponder the beauty of his character. God has a unique way of showing us love when it comes to his love and he constantly shows us that his love is superior to our love.

In fact his love is a mystery; so much so that the selfish person cannot comprehend it. A selfish person will wonder why love bad people so deeply, especially when there is a chance they will not love you in return. When we fall in love we want to do it with someone who will love us back but God showed loved to people without expectations. He asks for nothing in return. Most people respond with praise and acceptance of the Kingdom of God in their lives and others may take advantage of his love.

But God wants to love because that's who he is and he wants to lovingly restore the broken soul that has never learned about love, as well as the soul that has experience hatred.

He is the creator who gives men and women choices; and he lets men choose love, selfishness, or the world. I am unsure of where you stand but I choose love.

I choose love because it represents the truth and God's character has been tested and proven. He testifies that choosing him means that we are choosing to live above all the negative unloving things in the world around us.

He wants us to recognize how evil works but he does not want evil within us. Evil desires to hurt other people through words, actions, and thoughts but I can't speak for others but I want to love.

I want to live a life that is buried deep in his love. I believe that it is impossible for me to exhaust his love. I have made some horrible choices in life but his love has redeemed my time, circumstances, and life. I believe it is awesome that he tests us to ensure that we can handle his love.

The love of God has been my teacher and he has truly loved me. I desire that every man realize that abuse is not always being mean to a person but it is also abuse to say that you love someone so much that you overlook their nasty behavior. Both scenarios are a representation of not loving a person. Love corrects, love disciplines, and love doesn't hurt.

We must learn how to express love; and it is very important to show our children how to love by example.

Research shows that when we have physical contact with those we love we are creating a bond; and that bond is not easily broken. Children develop bonds with family and they learn how to imitate relationships.

Children who receive good words, kind and proper touching, and affirmations have healthy brain functions that fire off properly. The bonus to this is these children grow up healthy and become ready to demonstrate what they have learned at home.

Some parents who come from abusive backgrounds never learn how to show love and the people around them never feel loved by them because there is no expression of the love. Is it possible to love you by looking at you? Can I expect another person to just assume I love them? When we think about God and his love. It is something he showed and it is something he did. I watched a wife tell her husband, "Why don't you ever tell me you love me?" I was a little shocked at her because he cooked, he cleaned, he supported her. His actions said I love you but she wanted to hear it. Which is greater to you? Love is all about how the person treats you. Another woman can have a man who says "Baby I love you" a hundred times a day but he never cooks or helps her out. She carries all the burdens in the household. I think and believe God wants us to know that love is not saying it a hundred times it is in actions. You will know they love you by how they treat you.

When his or her love is still a feeling in the heart it can be deceptive to believe that this is the proper way to love someone. Real love is chemicals being released in the brain but real love also means that we make intelligent decisions every day towards the person we love. This means that love should be expressed in our actions. This is when we have entered into real love. As long as it is just the feelings it is at risked. Do not invest in feelings invest in someone who values you.

There are verbal and non-verbal ways to express our feelings. We can use compliments, showing of consideration, saying things such as I love you, or sending a sweet love letter, eye contact, sharing feelings, thoughtful actions, light touches, small favors without a word, all these things are actions and expressions of what we say or how we feel about the person.

When we share feelings and actions of love for someone we are creating a bond. When something becomes bonded it is hard to break apart. Do not bond with someone that tears you down. You want to bond with someone that brings you up.

From my experience with love; it has been my discoveries that love really do make us feel special. A bad love experience really can make you feel like the world is coming to an end.

I really enjoy the love stories in the movies as well as the fairy tales but those things do not teach us about love in everyday life.

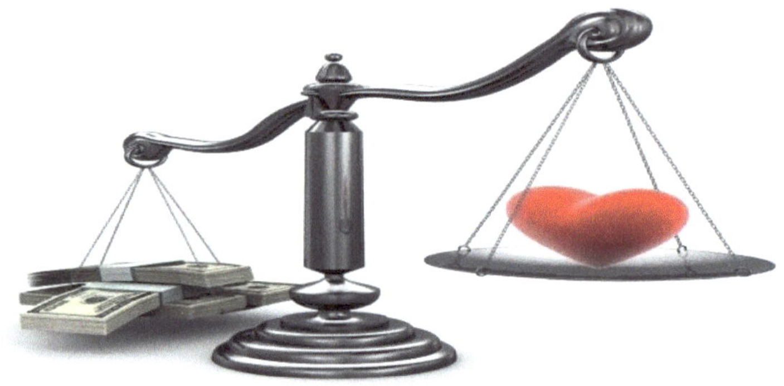

Research and studies have provided us with enough information in order to help us begin to think about our own definition of love. If we put it all together we know that when we fall in love, we idealize the individual and it is a natural thing to do; and by doing this we can begin to understand that when we idealize someone we see what we want to see about that person. It is very important to see the good so that we can stay in love with that person but it is not good to see only what we want to see. Some people say love is blind. Is it?

The Washington Post featured a very interesting article on, "The Brain on Love." According to the article all relationships change the brain. In fact brain scans have revealed that we have neural pathways that are set a blazed and a happy marriage have the power to relieve stress. Studies reveal that love is like a school; it is not any school but it is a tough school and we must remember that the studying is intense and the homework is hard.

The article also revealed that when we are burned by a lover, or rejected by a lover we experience a painful hurt all over the body; but in reality it is the "dorsal anterior cingulate cortex in the brain, it is located in the front of the collar part of the brain and it wraps around the corpus callosum, the bundle of nerve fibers zinging messages between the hemispheres that register both rejection and physical assault.

I have experienced rejection in love and it sucks. The pain is a natural feeling that hits the soul like a ton of bricks. I have discovered the cure and the grace and freedom that comes as a direct result of letting go and forgiving the person. Sometimes it is a blessing. If a person cannot match your love it is better to find someone that can.

Each instance of rejection happened to me because I was an unhealthy person and I associated with other unhealthy people. The concept is better understood through the saying show me who your friends are; and I will show you, who you are or who you will become. It is the idea that we surround ourselves with people that agree with us.

I learned at age thirty that I need to learn about love and I really messed up my love experiences in my twenties; I had many relationships in my life that were bad; and I was a bad person to be in relationship with.

When we met God we learn what love is and we stop the fantasy and stop creating ideals of love based upon negative experiences.

I have learned so much from my mistakes and I have discovered that everyone is worthy to be treated good no matter who we are. I have learned that we must first treat ourselves good if we expect others to treat us good.

I have made the decision to never settle for less. You can never be happy with a person whom you say you love but you hate the way they treat you. Love and abuse do not mix. It's vital to end the abuse because the brain needs healthy experiences; and we must allow ourselves to develop and grow in love.

I know that the past is over and it is not fun remembering the times we experienced heart breaks, bad romances, or the good or bad friendships along the way but for the sake of learning it is wise to learn from the experience. It is important to not to linger to long on past hurts but to learn from them in order to live a greater love life.

We can learn from the past mistakes in order to forgive others; I promise that the love journey is filled with discovery, growth, and learning!

The Future is better than the Past!

The latter shall be greater than the former. Sometimes the beginning of a thing starts off rocky. For example, my first experiences were very rocky; but I refuse to let my rocky beginning be my ending.

I always embrace hope and love. I believe that all things are possible with God. I am the person who cries during love stories and romantic endings. Do you like the beautiful endings of love stories where the King and Queen unit and conquer; or the prince and princess find true love despite the odds? I have always adored these fairy tale endings as a child and adult.

The greatest love story of all times is the story of Jesus Christ. His love surpasses anything I could ever image. His love for me has not only been my happy ending but it has taught me how to love the right way; and loving the right way is the result of knowing and learning about love from God.

I know that there are a lot of woman out there who may share my love for happy endings; and the good thing about this book is that love is positive and the focus is about creating a healthy love life.

I believe that our love lives can be better than the stories we see in the movies!

It is hard to start a great love life without confessing and admitting to any past sins and short comings. I had to admit to myself that I was defeated in my current love life. With that in mind I want to say that it was seven years ago when I waved my white flag during my prayer time. I was moving on from a very negative experience and I was very happy to be removed from the situation; I was relieved to be separated from the bad but at the same time I was hurt. So many negative things had taken place. It didn't matter who said what; or who did what but what mattered most to me was moving forward and learning how to never make the same mistake twice. At that time I wasn't old enough to understand the place that God had my heart in. I remember wanting to understand why things happened the way they did. I simply didn't get why my relationships were failing. God revealed to me that I didn't know how to show love. I had love in my heart. I am able to think about love but I struggle to show love. I was either super nice and you could do anything to me or I was really mean and guarded. I had to learn that I made bad choices in men.

I was down but at the same time I was lifted up because I had hope. I knew in my heart that I was young but I had a bright future. I begin to pray for God to teach me how to love.

It was important for me to not focus on the things that had taken place; it didn't matter if it was my fault or not, what matter to me was learning how to love.

In my inner most being I could feel God's sadness; and I could sense him reminding me of all the things he had told me to do in order to have a better relationship but I didn't obey the things that he told me. I learned very quickly that every relationship must work the way God designed it.

Lesson one was always remember the importance of choosing good people to be in relationship with. We have the power to choose and whatever we choose rather its good or bad we are the ones who have to live with the choice. I begin to feel frustration during this time because I thought to myself how could I choose good people if I was unhealthy. That drove me to seek God with all my heart because I didn't want to experience the same failure again.

People don't come into your life and wreck it. We make choices; and sometimes we realize we saw what we wanted to see in bad relationships.

If you have made bad choices like me I suggest you pray and ask God to help you with the choice to stay or leave because the relationship can be saved but it is a personal choice to make; most of us established relationships before we begin to serve God, and those choices were our choices.

It doesn't matter which category you fit in because God will change your life and help you discover his plan for life. He will work out every detail of our life in order to ensure that his will, will be done. No matter the situation have faith in God and trust his word.

I decided to become a winner. Today I am happy to report that I maintain a healthy love life; and I am committed to learning every day. I have learned so much. I am single. I date but I have healthy dating relationships. I have no more drama. Sometimes drama comes from that past negative relationship but I keep moving. A sour ex is something that can spoil your life. Run, run, run.

I decided to be the star in my own real life love story. As the star I get to create. I get to choose the person I will date, marry, and the friends I choose to associate with. I know that it may sound strange but a long time ago; I was so empty and needy for love. I looked like a beggar. I used to beg for love and moan and groan about how this person didn't love me, and that person didn't love me, and guess what, still today they still don't love me, but God became enough for me.

I was needy and my neediness could be seen in the way I carried myself, and people don't want to pour into a needy desperate person. Desperation makes a woman make bad choices in men. I am talking about the men who date multiple women at the same time. Some of them are not honest about their intentions. A desperate woman or man will try to make it work because a piece of man is better than not having a man. That's really sad.

I know that men and women go through similar and different issues, but guys sometimes have their mothers as their best friends and they can be alone and get comfort from their mothers while women typically go through alone. During these times the enemy can play with mind. I believe his goal is to try to convince the person that their failure is final; and that it's over for them and they might as well throw in the towel. But God wants us to be able to recognize and give love, seeking nothing in return. For example what is it to love someone who loves you back, but God desires for us to learn to love those who don't love us back? I promise you, it's so fulfilling.

Lesson II

I learned that God wants us to give love to others and he wants us to give it freely asking for nothing in return. We love because we are his children and he wants us to receive love from him instead of desiring a desperate love. If we receive love from him like a child needs love at home we become individuals who recognize real love and we will be able to choose people who are able to love us the right way and then we begin to attract love to us.

For example a person looking for love is seeking someone to meet their needs according to what they believe their needs are. A person who abides in God's love is a person who knows how to love and they will always attract love right back to them because they are ruling and reigning over the issues of the heart.

Once again I am the star of my love story and I must become healthy in order to attract healthy things into my life. For a long time I attracted the same type of drama and problems. I realized that the person and place changed but the issues remain the same.

I wondered why? I continuing to attract the same type of person. I learned from God that deep inside of me was an unhealthy heart; and my heart always seemed to be attracted to abusive unhealthy relationships.

Do you see any patterns in your love life? Have you encountered liars, cheaters, abusers, emotional abusive people, or physical abuse more than you wish to admit to? This type of treatment leaves devastating impacts on the heart.

You Are The Star!

The star is the leading person. The star of the story must have the right perception. The co-star and the star are somewhat equal but not completely equal. The star and the costar must go together like peanut and jelly; but the story must be led by the star and the star shines.

Sometimes family and friends might disapprove of a relationship because they feel like the star is being overshadow by the co-star.

Relationships should always make you better and not worst. If you have had bad relationships, it's not good to completely blame other people for all the faults; they carry some of the fault but it's always healthy to learn from these experiences and if you are perfect you don't have anything to learn; but if you analyze yourself and you discover that it takes two to make a bad relationship you can then forgive the person and God will bless you with wisdom and knowledge about love.

You will not only move forward but you will have the wisdom that comes from god and it will elevate you so that you do not make the same mistakes and that's when you can truly enjoy your life.

As the star of your love story, how do you view love? Let's think about our beliefs concerning love. This is important because we can measure love in different ways. For example:

- I use to believe that my relationships were all about me.

- I believed that a significant other is responsible for my happiness.

- I believed that I could be in a relationship without God.

- I believed that any person in relationship with me should be able to read my mind.

- I allowed my actions to be inspired by my emotions.

- I believed that I was perfect.

I believed all the wrong things. Right now I believe that every issue should be discussed; and God should be the center of the relationship and that means you have to marry a believer so that God can be in the middle.

Some people believe that love is sex, others believe that love consist of being showered with gifts, and money, while others believe love is passive and it never says anything that will offend them; right or wrong.

But the bible says that love is patient, it is not passive, love is kind, it is not easily provoked, a person who loves you will not be jealous of you and they will seek the best for you.

My unhealthy perception about love stopped me from experiencing love on a deeper level. God wanted to enlighten me about real love because God removed me from the darkness in order to help me experience his pure love.

The darkness in the world wants us to believe that loving others will cause us to be hurt. I am writing this book to testify that love never hurt me. People who loved me helped me to become a better person. People who reject love will eventually hurt people ignorantly. God desires that even that type of person can learn how to love.

Changing Perceptions

Right now take a few moments and think about how you perceive, receive, and give love. Secondly, I want you to think about the values and morals taught to you as a child. Lastly, I want you to think about how you measure love.

For example I have lots of values concerning love. I like taking time to think about my values concerning love because I like to measure where I am with love.

The bible reveals that God's love is measurable. It is very deep. As far as the heavens is from the earth. His love is a perfect love and my love tank increases every year.

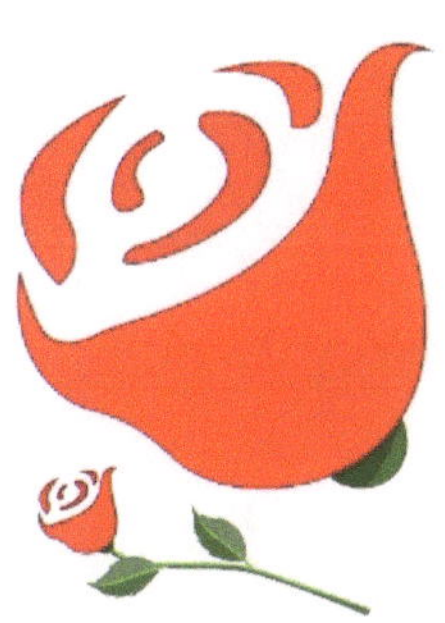

Measuring your tank means measuring, and analyzing personal love experiences; in order to determine how those experiences have cause you to love more or love less.

Sometimes bad experiences cause us to love less; and great experiences cause us to love more. Our love tank measurement reveals a lot about us; it determines if we have allowed negative experiences to affect how we love.

For example when my heart opened up to Jesus Christ my life changed. My mouth boldly declared him as my savior; and my love experience changed but my perception changed. I wanted God to love my unhealthy thoughts, lifestyle, and feel sorry for me but God took away my dirty garments and gave me the garment of praise, a garment of beauty, and a garment of health. He doesn't want us to hold on to the old thinking patterns.

Perception and experience will determine how we love others as well as what type of love we will experience.

I learned that it is unhealthy to view love through negative experiences. How other people treat you should never affect how you feel about yourself.

In the movie *The Grinch who stole Christmas;* the Grinch was not always a Grinch; in the movie starring Jim Carrey; the Grinch was a baby brought to town by the stork; he was green and different looking. The children made fun of him. His experiences with them made him feel like an outsider and he begin to develop an outsider mentally. He believed that if they rejected him than he would reject them by being detestable. In reality only 30% percent of the people rejected him and the other 70% actually liked him. The majority does not always win. Sometimes the cruel few win because the others do not have the courage to go against the cruel 30%.

In the end Cindy Lou Who's love, and acceptance for him caused him to love; and eventually he begins to love those that she loved. Her kindness turned him from Grinch who wanted to steal Christmas to the Grinch who restored Christmas. He was mean but her kindness melted his heart.

I have learned that the darkness in the world seeks to make people feel like they are so bad that nobody loves or likes them; as if there is something genetically wrong with a person and the effects is, that person is unable to be love, wanted, and they shall feel like they are less than others.

We must focus on our good experiences because God created every person with a desire and need for love and if we let the negative rule then we will miss out on love.

Once again, I know that some people have been blessed to have people in their life who have been great examples of love. I also know that some people have experience horrible situations. This brings us to lesson number III; love and truth go hand in hand.

Bad relationships are destructive relationships that counterfeit real love. These relationships are blinding because we may love the person but hate how the person treats you.

I am sure this idea is foreign to those who have a bundle of healthy relationships. For example a person can be in a relationship with a person who cheats, Abuses, and hurts them, and they just can't seem to get out the relationship. We shake our heads in dislike but remember relationship bonds begin in the beginning; this is another reminder about the importance of making good choices.

Of course anyone in a toxic relationship is living a lie and maybe somebody can convince them that the relationship lacks real love; but the person has to accept the fact that they are in a relationship with a destructive person. What will happen to you? Are you able to save them? The answer is you will be destroyed and God did not give us the power to save others. We can inspire and encourage but change is individual.

Real love is faithfulness, truth, and companionship; and this does not mean that temptation will not come. But your co-star loves you, and you love them, both of you will fight temptation in order to keep your love flame burning.

Real love will make a woman or man run from the sexy person on their job, because they can't stand the thought of losing you. If a person doesn't mind losing you than they don't need you. I refuse to be upset at any person who does not value me.

When I want to remember my value in relationships I think about money. If I put two hundred dollars and two cents in my wallet; and later on I discover that I only have one hundred dollars and one cent I will be very upset. I am going to chase and look for the one I value the most. I value that 100-dollar bill and honestly I may forget about the penny, but I am going to go through the whole house until I find the hundred-dollar bill. I believe that we all have value and it's not up to others to know our value but it's for us to know our value; and when a person doesn't mind losing you, you may be the penny in the relationship. Others see how much you value you by looking at what you permit into your life, despite your upbringing, and experiences.

Love!

Now, let us remove the idea, that love is how others have treated us. A bad experience doesn't mean you can't learn how to love. For example a boyfriend, husband, mother, or father may have treated you bad and affected your view of love; but this does not have to be the end of the story.

Love is patient, love is kind, it is not self-seeking, it is not boastful, and seeks not its own; and Love is an entity that should be viewed and measured by the true definition of love; and if we view love and express our feelings of love based upon how others have treated us then we will fail to experience true love. It's time to embrace the facts about love. We spend so much time determining how we love based upon how we been treated. We never think about how much power we have to learn how to love; and when we get the opportunity to experience love at a deeper level we learn that love has more to do with how you treat your man or woman. Today let us enter into the school of love; and instead of allowing other people to determine how we love we need to love because we know how.

For example, some women may have been in a relationship with a man that lied or cheated. Some move on but they say, I will never let that happen again, and so they become guarded or she transforms herself into the human lie detector. She can spot a liar a mile away; and she is determined to make sure that the next man earned her trust and commitment. The next man is paying the price for the last man. A man should never be judged based on a previous relationship. Just turn off the emotions and keep the brain in the front to make sure that he is worthy of your treasure.

Now the woman in the case study definitely has been mistreated, and she should feel the feelings of disappointment but a healthy woman understands the fact, that one man is not all men.

I wonder how many people let these experiences drive them instead of letting it go, and asking ourselves what attracted me to this person; we also need to pray to God to help us make better choices.

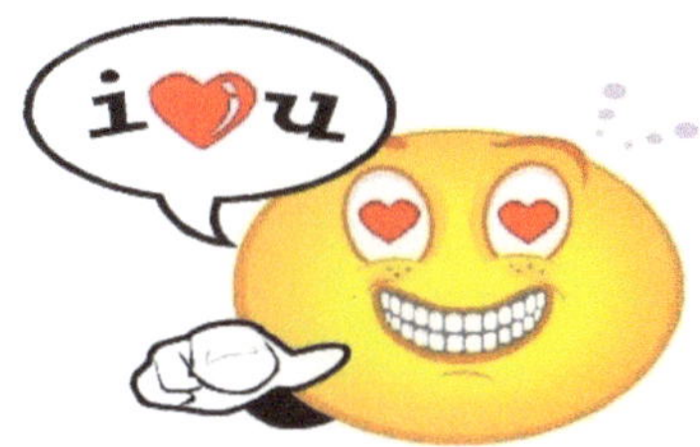

New relationships deserve fresh perspectives; because our love tank may have been emptied by the liar we met last month and today we have to have faith to believe God for a new experience.

I believe that it is important to look at ourselves no matter if the other person is at fault because for some reason we could be attracted to liars, abusers, or just maybe the behavior is the result of a response to bad behavior. People should never be our standard of love but our standard should come from God. He is the perfect lover. His love is pure and beautiful. On my journey to learning about love I discovered that I had a low measurement of love.

Taking Inventory

On a scale ranging from 1 to 100% where 1 is the lowest, and 100 the highest, I want you to measure your level of love. For example what would the people in your life rate your level of love. Write the rating, and explain. Be truthful.

____

____

____

____

____

____

____

My love measurement used to be 25%. Right now my love ability is 75%. I love my new rating; and I am determined to keep learning how to treat others the way I want to be treated and this makes a huge difference in the way I accept my friendships and associates. I am only willing to receive what I am ready to give out. If someone is offering me less than I am giving than I might not accept the offer. It has taken me a long time to realize and understand exactly what love is; but because I have experience the down side of love at a young age; right now I am at a stage in my life where I have a full love tank; and I want to spend it on a man whom I believe is worthy of my treasure.

My love tank is not full because of a person but it full because of God. I decided to trust his word and I truly believe that God hurts when we hurt; and sometimes in relationships we can get hurt because we lack the knowledge of love and we connect with others who do not know the source of Love, and that is God. Even though I have not met the man I want to spend it on yet, I am preparing myself to continue to grow in love so that I can make sure that I treat the man in my life; the way a man should be treated. I want to make sure that he is healthy and happy. Instead of watching love on TV; I want to star in my own love story. The movies and fairy tales are not bad examples but they only provide us with a limited view of relationships. I love a good love story on the big screen but in real life the story is longer and the characters are real people.

I always like to remember the law of attraction. The law of attraction excites me because we will always attract to us what we are. Getting married is beautiful but staying married takes time and a commitment to fall in love with the man who uncovers you and sees the value in you.

My testimony has layers of complexity. You have to get rid of your weaknesses because people can see them. I know that our world is very strange but it's true that the world enjoys magnifying and exploiting your weaknesses some people do it for a good laugh, others do it to make themselves feel better because they are in denial about their own weaknesses, or sometimes you will find that some people are just plain old mean. If you happen to be in an abusive relationship, pray and ask God to guide and lead you because God desires for us to know and receive love. We can also learn about love from family, friends, associates, and groups. It doesn't matter if we live in a community where love is visible or not, however every man, woman, and child have the opportunity to know love through God. A person who truly wants to experience love will forgive anyone who has fail to love them even those who mistreated them because they know Jesus Christ, and we know that, the people who hurt others are hurting themselves and they do not know God, or his love, because God is love, and we do know and recognize love because we know God. We do not have the power to dictate to others how they should treat us but we have the power to determine how we are going to treat others. Instead of fighting and hurting others we have to become an example and live inside out. Think about a person who have abused you, if you hang on to that, then that person lives in your mind. The healthy thing to do is give it over to God and forgive. We can then put ourselves in position to gain knowledge about any hurt or pain that happened to us. God will reveal or choose not to reveal information but we have to trust to him. We also get the opportunity to step back and discern and learn how we are to treat others; and that determines my expectations of who I let into my life. We will never have the opportunity to change the past but if we choose to love at a deeper level then we will get the opportunity to make sure that our new relationships will develop healthy and that they are based upon our new love foundations.

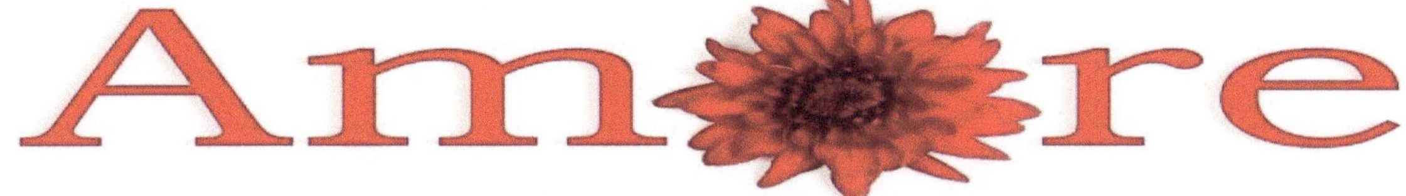

References

Louann Brizendine. (2014). Love, Sex, and the Male Brain. CNN. www.cnn.com

Thraybule, Linda. (2012). What Falling in Love Does to the Brain. Love Science. www.livescience.com

The Brain HQ "Your Brain in Love. Post it Science. www.brainhq.com

The National Washington Post. Love is in the mind, not the heart. www.washingtonpost.com

The Bible. The New King James Version, printed (2014).

The NIV Bible. NIV Translation.

Nakisha Marie Hercule

B.A Degree in English

MED degree in Education

I am a Christian, teacher, mother, writer, and graduate student. In my spare time I enjoy helping others achieve their dreams of writing.

I hope that this book has been a blessing to you because it has been a blessing to me.

I enjoyed writing this book, and I hope it fills your mind with knowledge, wisdom, and love, in order to build you up.

I learned at a very young age that love is complex. I didn't understand love in my twenties and it wasn't until I became old enough to believe in God that I learned what real love is.

I don't know about you but I want to love, love, and love some more because I know that my daughter is watching and learning from me.

Follow my blogs at beautygracestylelovenew.blogspot.com

favorablepublishing@gmail.com

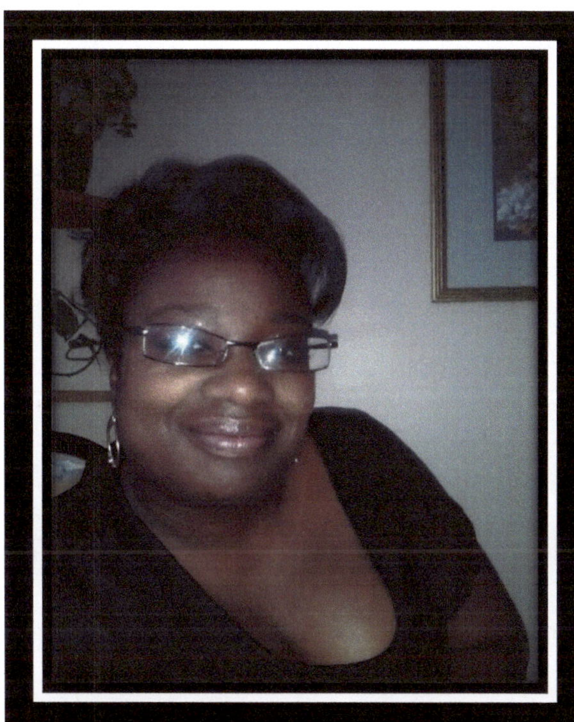
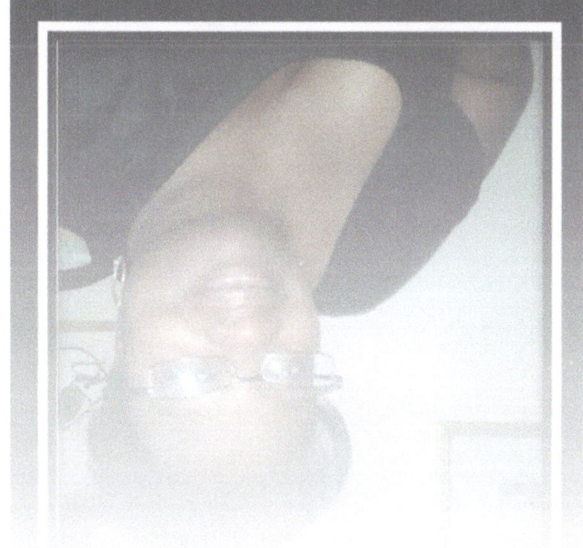

Love, Love, & More love

to you and yours!

Building Up Publishing Co.

www.ingramcontent.com/pod-product-compliance
Lightning Source LLC
Chambersburg PA
CBHW040049240726
48664CB00004B/1127